CW00570842

The Diabetic Cookbook for Beginners

The Beginners Guide to the Diabetes Diet with Tasty Recipes to Stay Healthy without Deprivation!

Kimberly Crooks

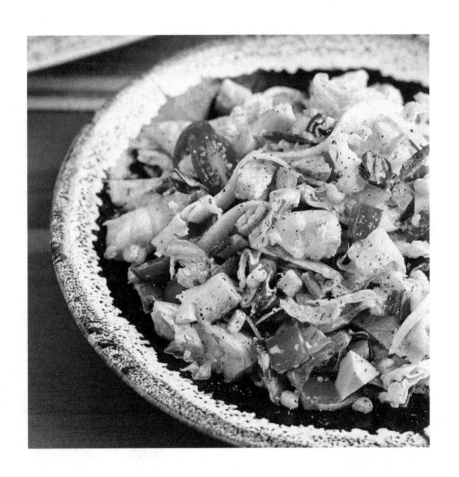

Table of Contents

The information in the following pages is broadly considered a truthful and accurate account of facts and as such, any inattention, use, or misuse of the information in question by the reader will render any resulting actions solely under their purview. There are no scenarios in which the publisher or the original author of this work can be in any fashion deemed liable for any hardship or damages that may befall them after undertaking information described herein.

Additionally, the information in the following pages is intended only for informational purposes and should thus be thought of as universal. As befitting its nature, it is presented without assurance regarding its prolonged validity or interim quality. Trademarks that are mentioned are done without written consent and can in no way be considered an endorsement from the trademark holder.

Introduction

Diabetes mellitus, commonly known just as diabetes, is a disease that affects our metabolism. The predominant characteristic of diabetes is an inability to create or utilize insulin, a hormone that moves sugar from our blood cells into the rest of our bodies' cells. This is crucial for us because we rely on that blood sugar to power our body and provide energy. High blood sugar, if left untreated, can lead to serious damage of our eyes, nerves, kidneys, and other major organs. There are two major types of diabetes, type 1 and type 2, with the latter being the most common of the two with over 90 percent of diabetics suffering from it (Centers for Disease Control and Prevention, 2019).

HOW DOES INSULIN WORK?

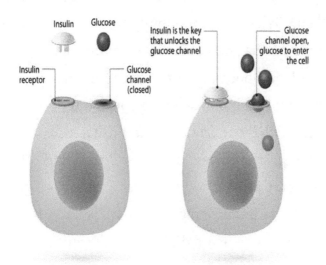

Type 1 diabetes is an autoimmune disease. In cases of type 1 diabetes, the immune system attacks cells in the pancreas responsible for insulin production. Although we are unsure what causes this reaction, many experts believe it is brought upon by a gene deficiency or by viral infections that may trigger the disease.

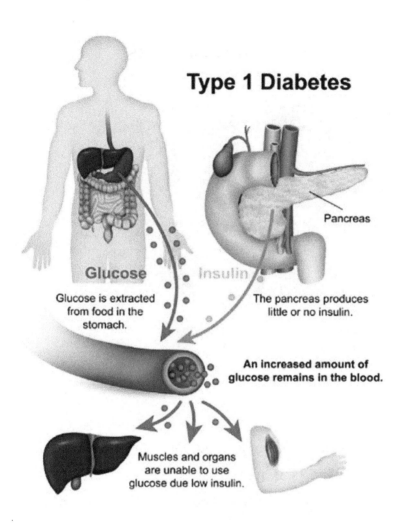

Type 1 Diabetes

Pancreas

Glucose

Insulin

Glucose is extracted from food in the stomach.

The pancreas produces little or no insulin.

An increased amount of glucose remains in the blood.

Muscles and organs are unable to use glucose due low insulin.

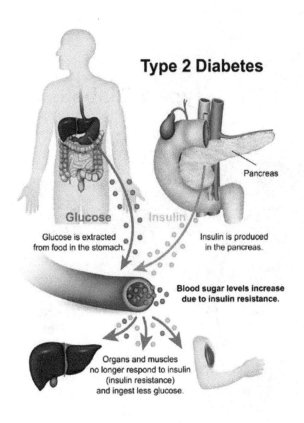

Type 2 Diabetes

Pancreas

Glucose   Insulin

Glucose is extracted
from food in the stomach.

Insulin is produced
in the pancreas.

**Blood sugar levels increase
due to insulin resistance.**

Organs and muscles
no longer respond to insulin
(insulin resistance)
and ingest less glucose.

Type 2 diabetes is a metabolic disorder, although research suggests it may warrant reclassification as an autoimmune disease as well. People who suffer from type 2 diabetes have a high resistance to insulin or an inability to produce enough insulin. Experts believe that type 2 diabetes is a result of a genetic predisposition in many people, which is further aggravated by obesity and other environmental triggers.

Diagnosis

Diabetes diagnosis has come incredibly far in the last few decades. Currently, there are two primary tests for diagnosing diabetes: the fasting plasma glucose (FPG) test and the hemoglobin A1c test.

The FPG test measures your blood sugar levels after an eight-hour fasting period; this helps to show if your body is processing glucose at a healthy rate.

The A1c test shows your blood sugar levels over the last three months. It does this by testing the amount of glucose being carried by the hemoglobin of your red blood cells. Hemoglobin has a lifespan of roughly three months; this allows us to test them to see how long they have been carrying their glucose for and how much they have.

Symptoms

In type 1 diabetes, the list of symptoms can be extensive with both serious and less obvious indicators. Below, I will list the most common symptoms as well as other potential complications of type 1 diabetes:

- **Excessive thirst:** Excessive thirst is one of the less noticeable indicators of type 1 diabetes. It is brought upon by high blood sugar (hyperglycemia).

- **Frequent urination:** Frequent urination is caused by your kidneys failing to process all of the glucose in your blood; this forces your body to attempt to flush out excess glucose through urinating.

- **Fatigue:** Fatigue in type 1 diabetes patients is caused by the body's inability to process glucose for energy.

- **Excessive hunger:** Those suffering from type 1 diabetes often have persistent hunger and increased appetites. This is because the body is desperate for glucose despite its inability to process it without insulin.

- **Cloudy or unclear vision:** Rapid fluctuations in blood sugar levels can lead to cloudy or blurred vision. Those suffering from untreated type 1 diabetes are unable to naturally control their blood sugar levels, making rapid fluctuations a very common occurrence.

- **Rapid weight loss:** Rapid weight loss is probably the most noticeable symptom of type 1 diabetes. As your body starves off glucose, it resorts to breaking down muscle and fat to sustain itself. This can lead to incredibly fast weight loss in type 1 diabetes cases.

SYMPTOMS OF TYPE 1 DIABETES

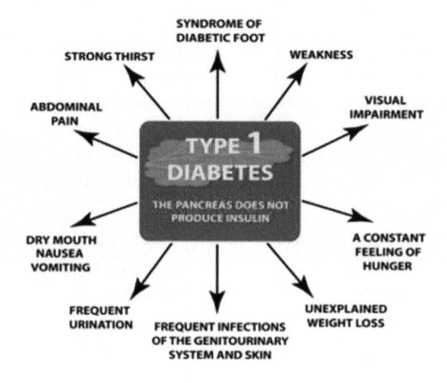

- **Ketoacidosis:** Ketoacidosis is a potentially deadly complication of untreated type 1 diabetes. In response to the lack of glucose being fed into your muscles and organs, your body starts breaking down your fat and muscle into an energy source called ketones, which can be burned without the need of insulin. Ketones are usually perfectly fine in normal amounts. But, when your body is starving, it may end up flooding itself with ketones in an attempt to fuel itself; the acidification of your blood that follows this influx of acid molecules may lead to more serious conditions, a coma, or death.

In cases of type 2 diabetes, the symptoms tend to be slower to develop, and they tend to be mild early on. Some early symptoms mimic type 1 diabetes and may include:

- **Excessive hunger:** Similar to type 1 diabetes, those of us with type 2 diabetes will feel constant hunger. Again, this is brought on by our bodies looking for fuel because of our inability to process glucose.

- **Fatigue and mental fog:** Depending on the severity of the insulin shortage in type 2 sufferers, they may feel physical fatigue and a mental fogginess during their average day.

- **Frequent urination:** Another symptom of both type 1 and 2 diabetes. Frequent urination is simply your body's way of attempting to rid itself of excess glucose.

- **Dry mouth and constant thirst:** It are unclear what causes dry mouth in diabetic sufferers, but it is tightly linked to high blood sugar levels. Constant thirst is brought on not only by a dry mouth but also by the dehydration that frequent urination causes.

SYMPTOMS OF TYPE 2 DIABETES

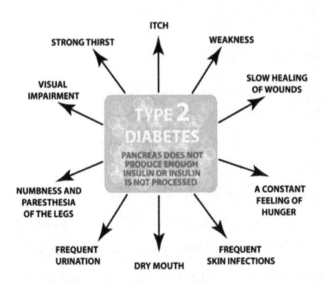

- **Itchy skin:** Itching of the skin, especially around the hands and feet, is a sign of polyneuropathy (diabetic nerve damage). As well as being a sign of potential nerve damage, itching can be a sign of high concentrations of cytokines circulating in your bloodstream; these are inflammatory molecules that can lead to itching. Cytokines are signaling proteins and hormonal regulators that are often released in high amounts before nerve damage.

As type 2 diabetes progresses and becomes more serious, the symptoms can become highly uncomfortable and dangerous. Some of these advanced symptoms include:

- **Slow healing of bruises, cuts, and abrasions:** Many people suffering from type 2 diabetes have impaired immune systems due to the lack of energy available to the body. As well as a lack of energy, many diabetics have slowed circulation brought upon by high blood glucose levels. Both of these factors lead to a much slower healing process and far greater risks of infection.

- **Yeast infections:** In women with type 2 diabetes, the chances of yeast infections are far higher than in non-diabetic women. This is due to high blood sugar levels and a lowered immune system response.

- **Neuropathy or numbness:** Long-term high blood sugar levels can lead to severe nerve damage in adults with diabetes. It is believed around 70 percent of people with type 2 diabetes have some form of neuropathy (Hoskins, 2020). Diabetic neuropathy is characterized by a numbness in the extremities, specifically around the feet and fingers.

- **Dark skin patches (acanthosis nigricans):** Some people with type 2 diabetes may have far above normal levels of insulin in their blood, as their body is unable to utilize it due to insulin resistance. This increase of insulin in the bloodstream can lead to some skin cells over reproducing and cause dark patches to form on the skin.

Complications

Severe complications of diabetes can be debilitating and deadly. Both type 1 and type 2 diabetes can lead to serious neurological, cardiovascular, and optical conditions. Some of the most common complications of advanced diabetes are as follows:

- **Heart attacks:** Diabetes is directly linked to a higher rate of heart attacks in adults. High blood glucose levels damage the cells and nerves around the heart and blood vessels over time, which can cause a plethora of heart diseases to form.

- **Cataracts:** People with diabetes have a nearly 60 percent greater chance of developing cataracts later in life if their diabetes is left unchecked (Diabetes.co.uk, 2019a). Doctors are unsure of the exact reason for cataracts forming at a higher rate in diabetes patients, but many believe it has to do with the lower amounts of glucose available to the cells powering our eyes.

- **Peripheral artery disease (PAD):** This is a very common diabetes and This causes decreased blood flow, which leads to serious issues in the lower legs, often resulting in amputation.

- **Diabetic nephropathy:** Diabetic nephropathy happens when high levels of blood glucose damage parts of your kidneys, which is responsible for filtering blood. This causes your kidneys to develop chronic kidney diseases and break down over time, leading to failure.

- **Glaucoma:** Diabetes can cause glaucoma in sufferers due to high blood sugar levels and this directly damages blood vessels in the eyes. When your body attempts to repair these vessels, it may cause glaucoma on the iris where the damage was caused.

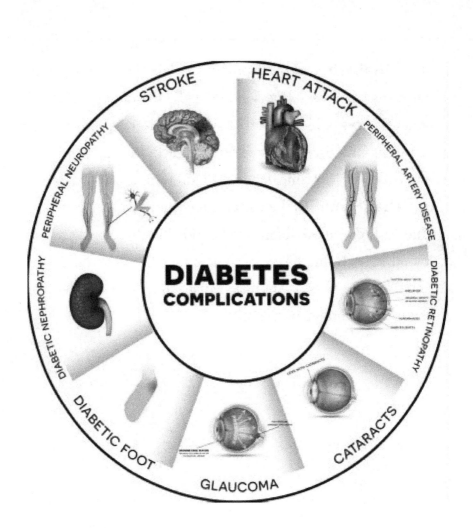

Treatment

Treatments for diabetes vary depending on the type, number, and severity of complications and health of the patient overall. Luckily, diabetes has been long studied by the medical community and, therefore, there is an abundance of resources and treatments available.

For type 1 diabetes, insulin supplements are essential. Type 1 diabetics rely on daily insulin injections; some prefer a costlier but easier-to-use insulin pump. Insulin needs in type 1 diabetics will vary throughout the day as they eat and exercise. This means many type 1 diabetics will regularly test their blood sugar levels to assess whether their insulin needs are being met.

Some type 1 diabetics develop insulin resistance after years of injections. This means that oral diabetes medication such as metformin is becoming increasingly more commonly prescribed to type 1 diabetics to help prevent insulin resistance.

Type 2 diabetes can be controlled without medication in some cases. Many type 2 diabetics can self-regulate their blood sugar levels through careful eating and light exercise. Most type 2 diabetics are recommended to stay on low-fat diets, which are high in fiber and healthy carbs.

Some type 2 diabetics do need medication. Unlike type 1, insulin is not nearly as commonly needed for type 2. But, some type 2 diabetics do need insulin to supplement the reduced amount their pancreas may provide.

The most common medication given to type 2 diabetics is metformin. This prescription drug helps lower blood glucose levels and improve insulin sensitivity. Other drugs prescribed to type 2 diabetics include sulfonylureas, thiazolidinediones, and meglitinides, which all help increase insulin production or sensitivity.

Diabetes
Blood Sugar Level

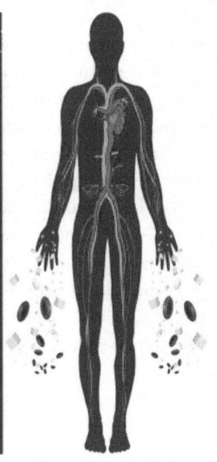

	HBA-1C Test Score	Mean Blood mg/dl	Glucose mmol/l
	14.0	380	21.1
	13.0	350	19.3
Action Suggested	12.0	315	17.4
	11.0	280	15.6
	10.0	250	13.7
	9.0	215	11.9
	8.0	180	10.0
Good	7.0	150	8.2
	6.0	115	6.3
Excellent	5.0	80	4.7
	4.0	50	2.6
	3.0	35	2.0

Very high
A little high to very high depending on patient
Maximum after meal in nondiabetics
Normal before meal in nondiabetics
Normal
Low
Extremely low

" The normal range of blood sugar
according to the glucose levels chart
is between 70 and 100 mg/dl "

10 Tips to Control Diabetes

- **Eat less salt:** Salt can increase your chances of having high blood pressure, which leads to increased chances of heart disease and stroke.

- **Replace sugar:** Replace sugar with zero calorie sweeteners. Cutting out sugar gives you much more control over your blood sugar levels.

- **Cut out alcohol:** Alcohol tends to be high in calories, and if drunk on an empty stomach with insulin medication, it can cause drastic drops in blood sugar.

- **Be physically active:** Physical activity lowers your risk of cardiovascular issues and increases your body's natural glucose burn rate.

- **Avoid saturated fats:** Saturated fats like butter and pastries can lead to high cholesterol and blood circulation issues.

- **Use canola or olive oil:** If you need to use oil in your cooking, use canola or olive oil. Both are high in beneficial fatty acids and monounsaturated fat.

- **Drink water:** Water is by far the healthiest drink you can have. Drinking water helps to regulate blood sugar and insulin levels.

- **Make sure you get enough vitamin D:** Vitamin D is a crucial vitamin for controlling blood sugar levels. Eat food high in this vitamin or ask your doctor about supplements.

- **Avoid processed food:** Processed foods tend to be high in vegetable oils, salt, refined grains, or other unhealthy additives.

- **Drink coffee and tea:** Not only are coffee and tea great hunger suppressants for dieters, but they contain important antioxidants that help with protecting cells.

Breakfast Recipes

Spicy Jalapeno Popper Deviled Eggs

Preparation Time: 5 minutes

Cooking Time: 5 minutes

Servings: 4

Ingredients

- 4 large whole eggs, hardboiled
- 2 tablespoons Keto-Friendly mayonnaise
- ¼ cup cheddar cheese, grated
- 2 slices bacon, cooked and crumbled
- 1 jalapeno, sliced

Directions:

1. Cut eggs in half, remove the yolk and put them in bowl
2. Lay egg whites on a platter
3. Mix in remaining ingredients and mash them with the egg yolks
4. Transfer yolk mix back to the egg whites
5. Serve and enjoy!

Nutrition:

Calories: 176

Fat: 14g

Carbohydrates: 0.7g

Protein: 10g

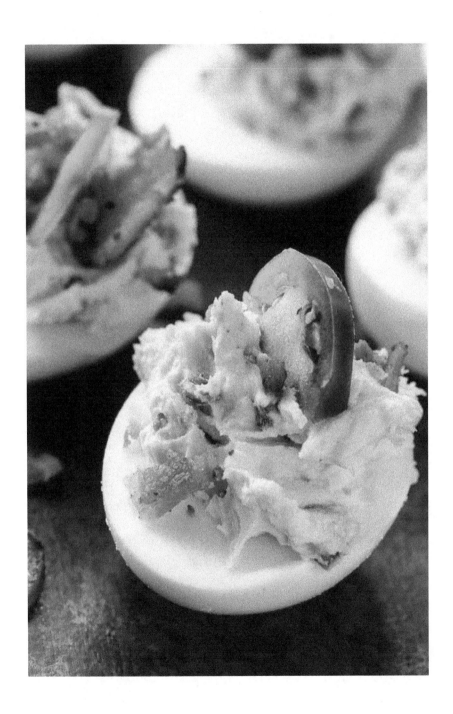

Lovely Porridge

Preparation Time: 15 minutes

Cooking Time: Nil

Servings: 2

Ingredients

- 2 tablespoons coconut flour
- 2 tablespoons vanilla protein powder
- 3 tablespoons Golden Flaxseed meal
- 1 and 1/2 cups almond milk, unsweetened
- Powdered erythritol

Directions:

1. Take a bowl and mix in flaxseed meal, protein powder, coconut flour and mix well
2. Add mix to the saucepan (placed over medium heat)
3. Add almond milk and stir, let the mixture thicken
4. Add your desired amount of sweetener and serve
5. Enjoy!

Nutrition:

Calories: 259

Fat: 13g

Carbohydrates: 5g

Protein: 16g

Salty Macadamia Chocolate Smoothie

Preparation Time: 5 minutes

Cooking Time: Nil

Servings: 1

Ingredients

- 2 tablespoons macadamia nuts, salted
- 1/3 cup chocolate whey protein powder, low carb
- 1 cup almond milk, unsweetened

Directions:

1. Add the listed ingredients to your blender and blend until you have a smooth mixture
2. Chill and enjoy it!

Nutrition:

Calories: 165

Fat: 2g

Carbohydrates: 1g

Protein: 12g

Basil and Tomato Baked Eggs

Preparation Time: 10 minutes

Cooking Time: 15 minutes

Servings: 4

Ingredients

- 1 garlic clove, minced
- 1 cup canned tomatoes
- ¼ cup fresh basil leaves, roughly chopped
- 1/2 teaspoon chili powder
- 1 tablespoon olive oil
- 4 whole eggs
- Salt and pepper to taste

Directions:

1. Preheat your oven to 375 degrees F
2. Take a small baking dish and grease with olive oil
3. Add garlic, basil, tomatoes chili, olive oil into a dish and stir
4. Crackdown eggs into a dish, keeping space between the two
5. Sprinkle the whole dish with salt and pepper
6. Place in oven and cook for 12 minutes until eggs are set and tomatoes are bubbling
7. Serve with basil on top

8. Enjoy!

Nutrition:

Calories: 235

Fat: 16g

Carbohydrates: 7g

Protein: 14g

Cinnamon and Coconut Porridge

Preparation Time: 5 minutes

Cooking Time: 5 minutes

Servings: 4

Ingredients

- 2 cups of water
- 1 cup 36% heavy cream
- 1/2 cup unsweetened dried coconut, shredded
- 2 tablespoons flaxseed meal
- 1 tablespoon butter
- 1 and 1/2 teaspoon stevia
- 1 teaspoon cinnamon
- Salt to taste
- Toppings as blueberries

Directions:

1. Add the listed ingredients to a small pot, mix well
2. Transfer pot to stove and place it over medium-low heat
3. Bring to mix to a slow boil
4. Stir well and remove the heat
5. Divide the mix into equal servings and let them sit for 10 minutes
6. Top with your desired toppings and enjoy!

Nutrition:

Calories: 171

Fat: 16g

Carbohydrates: 6g

Protein: 2g

An Omelet of Swiss chard

Preparation Time: 5 minutes

Cooking Time: 5 minutes

Servings: 4

Ingredients

- 4 eggs, lightly beaten
- 4 cups Swiss chard, sliced
- 2 tablespoons butter
- 1/2 teaspoon garlic salt
- Fresh pepper

Directions:

1. Take a non-stick frying pan and place it over medium-low heat
2. Once the butter melts, add Swiss chard and stir cook for 2 minutes
3. Pour egg into the pan and gently stir them into Swiss chard
4. Season with garlic salt and pepper
5. Cook for 2 minutes
6. Serve and enjoy!

Nutrition:

Calories: 260

Fat: 21g

Carbohydrates: 4g, Protein: 14g

Cheesy Low-Carb Omelet

Preparation Time: 5 minutes

Cooking Time: 5 minutes

Servings: 5

Ingredients

- 2 whole eggs
- 1 tablespoon water
- 1 tablespoon butter
- 3 thin slices salami
- 5 fresh basil leaves
- 5 thin slices, fresh ripe tomatoes
- 2 ounces fresh mozzarella cheese
- Salt and pepper as needed

Directions:

1. Take a small bowl and whisk in eggs and water
2. Take a non-stick Sauté pan and place it over medium heat, add butter and let it melt
3. Pour egg mixture and cook for 30 seconds
4. Spread salami slices on half of egg mix and top with cheese, tomatoes, basil slices
5. Season with salt and pepper according to your taste
6. Cook for 2 minutes and fold the egg with the empty half

7. Cover and cook on LOW for 1 minute

8. Serve and enjoy!

Nutrition:

- Calories: 451
- Fat: 36g
- Carbohydrates: 3g
- Protein:33g

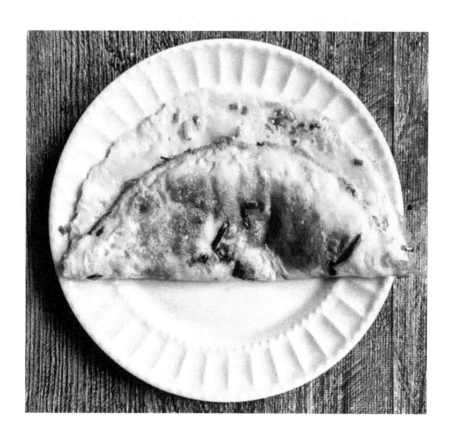

Yogurt and Kale Smoothie

Servings: 1

Preparation Time: 10 minutes

Ingredients:

- 1 cup whole milk yogurt
- 1 cup baby kale greens
- 1 pack stevia
- 1 tablespoon MCT oil
- 1 tablespoon sunflower seeds
- 1 cup of water

Directions:

1. Add listed ingredients to the blender
2. Blend until you have a smooth and creamy texture
3. Serve chilled and enjoy!

Nutrition:

Calories: 329

Fat: 26g

Carbohydrates: 15g

Protein: 11g

Bacon and Chicken Garlic Wrap

Preparation Time: 15 minutes

Cooking Time: 10 minutes

Servings: 4

Ingredients

- 1 chicken fillet, cut into small cubes
- 8-9 thin slices bacon, cut to fit cubes
- 6 garlic cloves, minced

Directions:

1. Preheat your oven to 400 degrees F
2. Line a baking tray with aluminum foil
3. Add minced garlic to a bowl and rub each chicken piece with it
4. Wrap bacon piece around each garlic chicken bite
5. Secure with toothpick
6. Transfer bites to the baking sheet, keeping a little bit of space between them
7. Bake for about 15-20 minutes until crispy
8. Serve and enjoy!

Nutrition:

- Calories: 260
- Fat: 19g
- Carbohydrates: 5g
- Protein: 22g

Grilled Chicken Platter

Preparation Time: 5 minutes

Cooking Time: 10 minutes

Servings: 6

Ingredients

- 3 large chicken breast, sliced half lengthwise
- 10-ounce spinach, frozen and drained
- 3-ounce mozzarella cheese, part-skim
- 1/2 a cup of roasted red peppers, cut in long strips
- 1 teaspoon of olive oil
- 2 garlic cloves, minced
- Salt and pepper as needed

Directions:

1. Preheat your oven to 400 degrees Fahrenheit
2. Slice 3 chicken breast lengthwise
3. Take a non-stick pan and grease with cooking spray
4. Bake for 2-3 minutes each side
5. Take another skillet and cook spinach and garlic in oil for 3 minutes
6. Place chicken on an oven pan and top with spinach, roasted peppers, and mozzarella
7. Bake until the cheese melted

8. Enjoy!

Nutrition:

Calories: 195

Fat: 7g

Net Carbohydrates: 3g

Protein: 30g

Parsley Chicken Breast

Preparation Time: 10 minutes

Cooking Time: 40 minutes

Servings: 4

Ingredients

- 1 tablespoon dry parsley
- 1 tablespoon dry basil
- 4 chicken breast halves, boneless and skinless
- 1/2 teaspoon salt
- 1/2 teaspoon red pepper flakes, crushed
- 2 tomatoes, sliced

Directions:

1. Preheat your oven to 350 degrees F
2. Take a 9x13 inch baking dish and grease it up with cooking spray
3. Sprinkle 1 tablespoon of parsley, 1 teaspoon of basil and spread the mixture over your baking dish
4. Arrange the chicken breast halves over the dish and sprinkle garlic slices on top
5. Take a small bowl and add 1 teaspoon parsley, 1 teaspoon of basil, salt, basil, red pepper and mix well. Pour the mixture over the chicken breast

6. Top with tomato slices and cover, bake for 25 minutes
7. Remove the cover and bake for 15 minutes more
8. Serve and enjoy!

Nutrition:

Calories: 150

Fat: 4g

Carbohydrates: 4g

Protein: 25g

Mustard Chicken

Preparation Time: 10 minutes

Cooking Time: 40 minutes

Servings: 4

Ingredients

- 4 chicken breasts
- 1/2 cup chicken broth
- 3-4 tablespoons mustard
- 3 tablespoons olive oil
- 1 teaspoon paprika
- 1 teaspoon chili powder
- 1 teaspoon garlic powder

Directions:

1. Take a small bowl and mix mustard, olive oil, paprika, chicken broth, garlic powder, chicken broth, and chili
2. Add chicken breast and marinate for 30 minutes
3. Take a lined baking sheet and arrange the chicken
4. Bake for 35 minutes at 375 degrees Fahrenheit
5. Serve and enjoy!

Nutrition:

Calories: 531

Fat: 23g

Carbohydrates: 10g

Protein: 64g

Balsamic Chicken

Preparation Time: 10 minutes

Cooking Time: 25 minutes

Servings: 6

Ingredients

- 6 chicken breast halves, skinless and boneless
- 1 teaspoon garlic salt
- Ground black pepper
- 2 tablespoons olive oil
- 1 onion, thinly sliced
- 14 and 1/2 ounces tomatoes, diced
- 1/2 cup balsamic vinegar
- 1 teaspoon dried basil
- 1 teaspoon dried oregano
- 1 teaspoon dried rosemary
- 1/2 teaspoon dried thyme

Directions:

1. Season both sides of your chicken breasts thoroughly with pepper and garlic salt
2. Take a skillet and place it over medium heat
3. Add some oil and cook your seasoned chicken for 3-4 minutes per side until the breasts are nicely browned

4. Add some onion and cook for another 3-4 minutes until the onions are browned

5. Pour the diced up tomatoes and balsamic vinegar over your chicken and season with some rosemary, basil, thyme, and rosemary

6. Simmer the chicken for about 15 minutes until they are no longer pink

7. Take an instant-read thermometer and check if the internal temperature gives a reading of 165 degrees Fahrenheit

8. If yes, then you are good to go!

Nutrition:

Calories: 196

Fat: 7g

Carbohydrates: 7g

Protein: 23g

Greek Chicken Breast

Preparation Time: 10 minutes

Cooking Time: 25 minutes

Servings: 4

Ingredients

- 4 chicken breast halves, skinless and boneless
- 1 cup extra virgin olive oil
- 1 lemon, juiced
- 2 teaspoons garlic, crushed
- 1 and 1/2 teaspoons black pepper
- 1/3 teaspoon paprika

Directions:

1. Cut 3 slits in the chicken breast
2. Take a small bowl and whisk in olive oil, salt, lemon juice, garlic, paprika, pepper and whisk for 30 seconds
3. Place chicken in a large bowl and pour marinade
4. Rub the marinade all over using your hand
5. Refrigerate overnight
6. Pre-heat grill to medium heat and oil the grate
7. Cook chicken in the grill until center is no longer pink
8. Serve and enjoy!

Nutrition:

Calories: 644

Fat: 57g

Carbohydrates: 2g

Protein: 27g

Chipotle Lettuce Chicken

Preparation Time: 10 minutes

Cooking Time: 25 minutes

Servings: 6

Ingredients

- 1 pound chicken breast, cut into strips
- Splash of olive oil
- 1 red onion, finely sliced
- 14 ounces tomatoes
- 1 teaspoon chipotle, chopped
- 1/2 teaspoon cumin
- Pinch of sugar
- Lettuce as needed
- Fresh coriander leaves
- Jalapeno chilies, sliced
- Fresh tomato slices for garnish
- Lime wedges

Directions:

1. Take a non-stick frying pan and place it over medium heat
2. Add oil and heat it up
3. Add chicken and cook until brown
4. Keep the chicken on the side

5. Add tomatoes, sugar, chipotle, cumin to the same pan and simmer for 25 minutes until you have a nice sauce
6. Add chicken into the sauce and cook for 5 minutes
7. Transfer the mix to another place
8. Use lettuce wraps to take a portion of the mixture and serve with a squeeze of lemon
9. Enjoy!

Nutrition:

Calories: 332

Fat: 15g

Carbohydrates: 13g

Protein: 34g

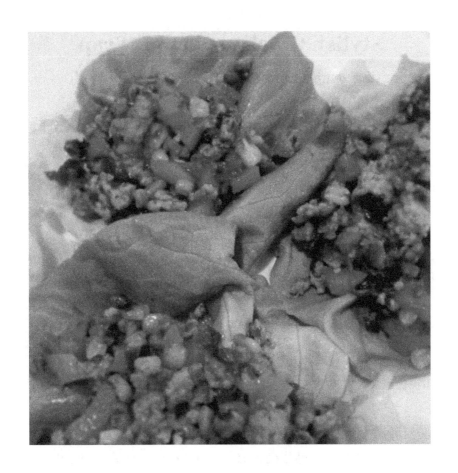

Stylish Chicken-Bacon Wrap

Preparation Time: 5 minutes

Cooking Time: 50 minutes

Servings: 3

Ingredients

- 8 ounces lean chicken breast
- 6 bacon slices
- 3 ounces shredded cheese
- 4 slices ham
- Directions:

1. Cut chicken breast into bite-sized portions
2. Transfer shredded cheese onto ham slices
3. Roll up chicken breast and ham slices in bacon slices
4. Take a skillet and place it over medium heat
5. Add olive oil and brown bacon for a while
6. Remove rolls and transfer to your oven
7. Bake for 45 minutes at 325 degrees F
8. Serve and enjoy!

Nutrition:

Calories: 275

Fat: 11g

Carbohydrates: 0.5g

Protein: 40g

Healthy Cottage Cheese Pancakes

Preparation Time: 10 minutes

Cooking Time: 15

Servings: 1

Ingredients:

- 1/2 cup of Cottage cheese (low-fat)

- 1/3 cup (approx. 2 egg whites) Egg whites

- ¼ cup of Oats

- 1 teaspoon of Vanilla extract

- Olive oil cooking spray

- 1 tablespoon of Stevia (raw)

- Berries or sugar-free jam (optional)

Directions:

1. Begin by taking a food blender and adding in the egg whites and cottage cheese. Also add in the vanilla extract, a pinch of stevia, and oats. Palpitate until the consistency is well smooth.

2. Get a nonstick pan and oil it nicely with the cooking spray. Position the pan on low heat.

3. After it has been heated, scoop out half of the batter and pour it on the pan. Cook for about 21/2 minutes on each side.

4. Position the cooked pancakes on a serving plate and cover with sugar-free jam or berries.

Nutrition: Calories: 205 calories per serving Fat – 1.5 g, Protein – 24.5 g, Carbohydrates – 19 g

Avocado Lemon Toast

Preparation Time: 10 minutes

Cooking Time: 13 minutes

Servings: 2

Ingredients:

- Whole-grain bread – 2 slices

- Fresh cilantro (chopped) – 2 tablespoons

- Lemon zest – ¼ teaspoon

- Fine sea salt – 1 pinch

Directions:

1. Begin by getting a medium-sized mixing bowl and adding in the avocado. Make use of a fork to crush it properly.

2. Then, add in the cilantro, lemon zest, lemon juice, sea salt, and cayenne pepper. Mix well until combined.

3. Toast the bread slices in a toaster until golden brown. It should take about 3 minutes.

4. Top the toasted bread slices with the avocado mixture and finalize by drizzling with chia seeds.

Nutrition:

- Calories: 72 calories per serving

- Protein – 3.6 g

- Avocado – 1/2

- Fresh lemon juice – 1 teaspoon

- Cayenne pepper – 1 pinch

- Chia seeds – ¼ teaspoon

- Fat – 1.2 g

- Carbohydrates – 11.6 g

Healthy Baked Eggs

Preparation Time: 10 minutes

Cooking Time: 1 hour

Servings: 6

Ingredients:

- Olive oil – 1 tablespoon

- Garlic – 2 cloves

- Eggs – 8 large

- Sea salt – 1/2 teaspoon

- Shredded mozzarella cheese (medium-fat) – 3 cups

- Olive oil spray

- Onion (chopped) – 1 medium

- Spinach leaves – 8 ounces

- Half-and-half – 1 cup

- Black pepper – 1 teaspoon

- Feta cheese – 1/2 cup

Directions:

1. Begin by heating the oven to 375F.

2. Get a glass baking dish and grease it with olive oil spray. Arrange aside.

3. Now take a nonstick pan and pour in the olive oil. Position the pan on allows heat and allows it heat.

4. Immediately you are done, toss in the garlic, spinach, and onion. Prepare for about 5 minutes. Arrange aside.

5. You can now Get a large mixing bowl and add in the half, eggs, pepper, and salt. Whisk thoroughly to combine.

6. Put in the feta cheese and chopped mozzarella cheese (reserve 1/2 cup of mozzarella cheese for later).

7. Put the egg mixture and prepared spinach to the prepared glass baking dish. Blend well to combine. Drizzle the reserved cheese over the top.

8. Bake the egg mix for about 45 minutes.

9. Extract the baking dish from the oven and allow it to stand for 10 minutes.

10. Dice and serve!

Nutrition:

Calories: 323 calories per serving

Fat – 22.3 g

Protein – 22.6 g

Carbohydrates – 7.9 g

Quick Low-Carb Oatmeal

Preparation Time: 10 minutes

Cooking Time: 15 minutes

Servings: 2

Ingredients:

- Almond flour – 1/2 cup

- Flax meal – 2 tablespoons

- Cinnamon (ground) – 1 teaspoon

- Almond milk (unsweetened) – 11/2 cups

- Salt – as per taste

- Chia seeds – 2 tablespoons

- Liquid stevia – 10 – 15 drops

- Vanilla extract – 1 teaspoon

Directions:

1. Begin by taking a large mixing bowl and adding in the coconut flour, almond flour, ground cinnamon, flax seed powder, and chia seeds. Mix properly to combine.

2. Position a stockpot on a low heat and add in the dry ingredients. Also add in the liquid stevia, vanilla extract, and almond milk. Mix well to combine.

3. Prepare the flour and almond milk for about 4 minutes. Add salt if needed.

4. Move the oatmeal to a serving bowl and top with nuts, seeds, and pure and neat berries.

Nutrition:

Calories: calories per serving

Protein – 11.7 g

Fat – 24.3 g

Carbohydrates – 16.7 g

Tofu and Vegetable Scramble

Preparation Time: 10 minutes

Cooking Time: 15 minutes

Servings: 2

Ingredients:

- Firm tofu (drained) – 16 ounces

- Sea salt – 1/2 teaspoon

- Garlic powder – 1 teaspoon

- Fresh coriander – for garnishing

- Red onion – 1/2 medium

- Cumin powder – 1 teaspoon

- Lemon juice – for topping

- Green bell pepper – 1 medium

- Garlic powder – 1 teaspoon

- Fresh coriander – for garnishing

- Red onion – 1/2 medium

- Cumin powder – 1 teaspoon

- Lemon juice – for topping

Directions:

1. Begin by preparing the ingredients. For this, you are to extract the seeds of the tomato and green bell pepper. Shred the onion, bell pepper, and tomato into small cubes.

2. Get a small mixing bowl and position the fairly hard tofu inside it. Make use of your hands to break the fairly hard tofu. Arrange aside.

3. Get a nonstick pan and add in the onion, tomato, and bell pepper. Mix and cook for about 3 minutes.

4. Put the somewhat hard crumbled tofu to the pan and combine well.

5. Get a small bowl and put in the water, turmeric, garlic powder, cumin powder, and chili powder. Combine well and stream it over the tofu and vegetable mixture.

6. Allow the tofu and vegetable crumble cook with seasoning for 5 minutes. Continuously stir so that the pan is not holding the ingredients.

Drizzle the tofu scramble with chili flakes and salt. Combine well.

7. Transfer the prepared scramble to a serving bowl and give it a proper spray of lemon juice.

8. Finalize by garnishing with pure and neat coriander. Serve while hot!

Nutritional Information:

Calories: 238 calories per serving

Carbohydrates – 16.6 g

Fat – 11 g

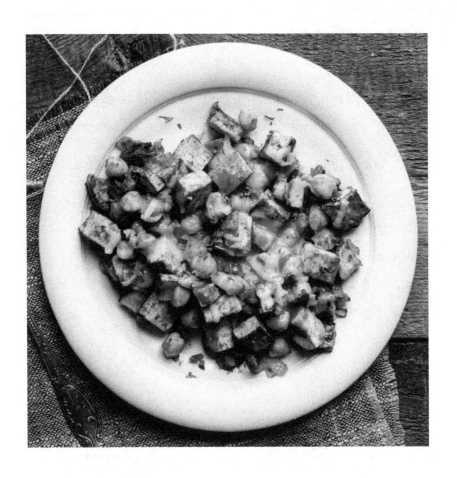

Breakfast Smoothie Bowl with Fresh Berries

Preparation Time: 10 minutes

Cooking Time: 5 minutes

Servings: 2

Ingredients:

- Almond milk (unsweetened) – 1/2 cup

- Psyllium husk powder – 1/2 teaspoon

- Strawberries (chopped) – 2 ounces

- Coconut oil – 1 tablespoon

- Crushed ice – 3 cups

- Liquid stevia – 5 to 10 drops

- Pea protein powder – 1/3 cup

Directions:

1. Begin by taking a blender and adding in the mashed ice cubes. Allow them to rest for about 30 seconds.

2. Then put in the almond milk, shredded strawberries, pea protein powder, psyllium husk powder, coconut oil, and liquid stevia. Blend well until it turns into a smooth and creamy puree.

3. Vacant the prepared smoothie into 2 glasses.

4. Cover with coconut flakes and pure and neat strawberries.

Nutrition:

Calories: 166 calories per serving

Fat – 9.2 g

Carbohydrates – 4.1 g

Protein – 17.6 g

Chia and Coconut Pudding

Preparation Time: 10 minutes

Cooking Time: 5 minutes

Servings: 2

Ingredients:

- Light coconut milk – 7 ounces

- Liquid stevia – 3 to 4 drops

- Kiwi – 1

- Chia seeds – ¼ cup

- Clementine – 1

- Shredded coconut (unsweetened)

Directions:

1. Begin by getting a mixing bowl and putting in the light coconut milk. Set in the liquid stevia to sweeten the milk. Combine well.

2. Put the chia seeds to the milk and whisk until well-combined. Arrange aside.

3. Scrape the clementine and carefully extract the skin from the wedges. Leave aside.

4. Also, scrape the kiwi and dice it into small pieces.

5. Get a glass vessel and gather the pudding. For this, position the fruits at the bottom of the jar; then put a dollop of chia pudding. Then spray the fruits and then put another layer of chia pudding.

6. Finalize by garnishing with the rest of the fruits and chopped coconut.

Nutrition:

Calories: 201 calories per serving

Protein – 5.4 g

Fat – 10 g

Carbohydrates – 22.8 g

Tomato and Zucchini Sauté

Preparation Time: 10 minutes

Cooking Time: 43 minutes

Servings: 6

Ingredients:

- Vegetable oil – 1 tablespoon

- Tomatoes (chopped) – 2

- Green bell pepper (chopped) – 1

- Black pepper (freshly ground) – as per taste

- Onion (sliced) – 1

- Zucchini (peeled) – 2 pounds and cut into 1-inch-thick slices

- Salt – as per taste

- Uncooked white rice – ¼ cup

Directions:

1. Begin by getting a nonstick pan and putting it over low heat. Stream in the oil and allow it to heat through.

Put in the onions and sauté for about 3 minutes.

2. Then pour in the zucchini and green peppers. Mix well and spice with black pepper and salt.

3. Reduce the heat and cover the pan with a lid. Allow the veggies cook on low for 5 minutes.

4. While you're done, put in the water and rice. Place the lid back on and cook on low for 20 minutes.

Nutrition:

Calories: 94 calories per serving

Fat – 2.8 g

Protein – 3.2 g

Carbohydrates – 16.1 g

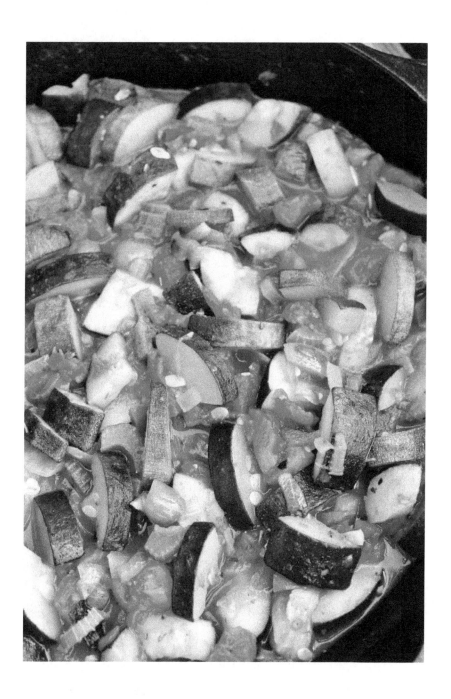

Steamed Kale with Mediterranean Dressing

Preparation Time: 10 minutes

Cooking Time: 25 minutes

Servings: 6

Ingredients:

- Kale (chopped) – 12 cups

- Olive oil – 1 tablespoon

- Soy sauce – 1 teaspoon

- Pepper (freshly ground) – as per taste

- Lemon juice – 2 tablespoons

- Garlic (minced) – 1 tablespoon

- Salt – as per taste

Directions:

1. Get a gas steamer or an electric steamer and fill the bottom pan with water. If making use of a gas steamer, position it on high heat. Making use of an electric steamer, place it on the highest setting.

---

2. Immediately the water comes to a boil, put in the shredded kale and cover with a lid. Boil for about 8 minutes. The kale should be tender by now.

3. During the kale is boiling, take a big mixing bowl and put in the olive oil, lemon juice, soy sauce, garlic, pepper, and salt. Whisk well to mix.

4. Now toss in the steamed kale and carefully enclose into the dressing. Be assured the kale is well-coated.

5. Serve while it's hot!

Nutrition:

Calories: 91 calories per serving

Fat – 3.5 g

Protein – 4.6 g

Carbohydrates – 14.5 g

Healthy Carrot Muffins

Preparation Time: 10 minutes

Cooking Time: 40 minutes

Servings: 8

Ingredients:

Dry ingredients

- Tapioca starch – ¼ cup

- Baking soda – 1 teaspoon

- Cinnamon – 1 tablespoon

- Cloves – ¼ teaspoon

- Wet ingredients

- Vanilla extract – 1 teaspoon

- Water – 11/2 cups

- Carrots (shredded) – 11/2 cups

- Almond flour – 1¾ cups

- Granulated sweetener of choice – 1/2 cup

- Baking powder – 1 teaspoon

- Nutmeg – 1 teaspoon

- Salt – 1 teaspoon

- Coconut oil – 1/3 cup

- Flax meal – 4 tablespoons

- Banana (mashed) – 1 medium

Directions:

1. Begin by heating the oven to 350F.

2. Get a muffin tray and position paper cups in all the moulds. Arrange aside.

3. Get a small glass bowl and put half a cup of water and flax meal. Allow this rest for about 5 minutes. Your flax egg is prepared.

4. Get a large mixing bowl and put in the almond flour, tapioca starch, granulated sugar, baking soda, baking powder, cinnamon, nutmeg, cloves, and salt. Mix well to combine.

5. Conform a well in the middle of the flour mixture and stream in the coconut oil, vanilla

extract, and flax egg. Mix well to conform a mushy dough.

Then put in the chopped carrots and mashed banana. Mix until well-combined.

6. Make use of a spoon to scoop out an equal amount of mixture into 8 muffin cups.

7. Position the muffin tray in the oven and allow it to bake for about 40 minutes.

8. Extract the tray from the microwave and allow the muffins to stand for about 10 minutes.

9. Extract the muffin cups from the tray and allow them to chill until they reach room degree of hotness and coldness.

10. Serve and enjoy!

Nutrition:

Calories: 189 calories per serving

Fat – 13.9 g

Protein – 3.8 g

Carbohydrates – 17.3 g

Vegetable Noodles Stir-Fry

Preparation Time: 10 minutes

Cooking Time: 40 minutes

Servings: 4

Ingredients:

- White sweet potato – 1 pound

- Zucchini – 8 ounces

- Garlic cloves (finely chopped) – 2 large

- Vegetable broth – 2 tablespoons

- Salt – as per taste

- Carrots – 8 ounces

- Shallot (finely chopped) – 1

- Red chili (finely chopped) – 1

- Olive oil – 1 tablespoon

- Pepper – as per taste

Directions:

1. Begin by scrapping the carrots and sweet potato. Make Use a spiralizer to make noodles out of the sweet potato and carrots.

2. Rinse the zucchini thoroughly and spiralize it as well.

3. Get a large skillet and position it on a high flame. Stream in the vegetable broth and allow it to come to a boil.

4. Toss in the spiralized sweet potato and carrots. Then put in the chili, garlic, and shallots. Stir everything using tongs and cook for some minutes.

5. Transfer the vegetable noodles into a serving platter and generously spice with pepper and salt.

6. Finalize by sprinkling olive oil over the noodles. Serve while hot!

Nutrition:

Calories: 169 calories per serving

Fat – 3.7 g

Protein – 3.6 g

Carbohydrates – 31.2 g

Berry-oat breakfast bars

Preparation time: 10 minutes

Cooking time: 25 minutes

Servings: 12

Ingredients:

- 2 cups fresh raspberries or blueberries

- 2 tablespoons sugar

- 2 tablespoons freshly squeezed lemon juice

- 1 tablespoon cornstarch

- 11/2 cups rolled oats

- 1/2 cup whole-wheat flour

- 1/2 cup walnuts

- ¼ cup chia seeds

- ¼ cup extra-virgin olive oil

- ¼ cup honey

- 1 large egg

Directions:

1. Preheat the oven to 350f.

2. In a small saucepan over medium heat, stir together the berries, sugar, lemon juice, and cornstarch. Bring to a simmer. Reduce the heat and simmer for 2 to 3 minutes, until the mixture thickens.

3. In a food processor or high-speed blender, combine the oats, flour, walnuts, and chia seeds. Process until powdered. Add the olive oil, honey, and egg. Pulse a few more times, until well combined. Press half of the mixture into a 9-inch square baking dish.

4. Spread the berry filling over the oat mixture. Add the remaining oat mixture on top of the berries. Bake for 25 minutes, until browned.

5. Let cool completely, cut into 12 pieces, and serve. Store in a covered container for up to 5 days.

Nutrition: calories: 201; total fat: 10g; saturated fat: 1g; protein: 5g; carbs: 26g; sugar: 9g; fiber: 5g; cholesterol: 16mg; sodium: 8mg

30 minutes or less • nut free • vegetarian

Whole-grain breakfast cookies

Preparation time: 20 minutes

Cooking time: 10 minutes

Servings: 18 cookies

Ingredients:

- 2 cups rolled oats

- 1/2 cup whole-wheat flour

- ¼ cup ground flaxseed

- 1 teaspoon baking powder

- 1 cup unsweetened applesauce

- 2 large eggs

- 2 tablespoons vegetable oil

- 2 teaspoons vanilla extract

- 1 teaspoon ground cinnamon

- 1/2 cup dried cherries

- ¼ cup unsweetened shredded coconut

- 2 ounces dark chocolate, chopped

Directions:

1. Preheat the oven to 350f.

2. In a large bowl, combine the oats, flour, flaxseed, and baking powder. Stir well to mix.

3. In a medium bowl, whisk the applesauce, eggs, vegetable oil, vanilla, and cinnamon. Pour the wet mixture into the dry mixture, and stir until just combined.

4. Fold in the cherries, coconut, and chocolate. Drop tablespoon-size balls of dough onto a baking sheet. Bake for 10 to 12 minutes, until browned and cooked through.

5. Let cool for about 3 minutes, remove from the baking sheet, and cool completely before serving. Store in an airtight container for up to 1 week.

Nutrition: calories: 136; total fat: 7g; saturated fat: 3g; protein: 4g; carbs: 14g; sugar: 4g; fiber: 3g; cholesterol: 21mg; sodium: 11mg

Blueberry breakfast cake

Preparation time: 15 minutes

Cooking time: 45 minutes

Servings: 12

Ingredients:

For the topping

- ¼ cup finely chopped walnuts

- 1/2 teaspoon ground cinnamon

- 2 tablespoons butter, chopped into small pieces

- 2 tablespoons sugar

For the cake

- Nonstick cooking spray

- 1 cup whole-wheat pastry flour

- 1 cup oat flour

- ¼ cup sugar

- 2 teaspoons baking powder

- 1 large egg, beaten

- 1/2 cup skim milk

- 2 tablespoons butter, melted

- 1 teaspoon grated lemon peel

- 2 cups fresh or frozen blueberries

Directions:

To make the topping

In a small bowl, stir together the walnuts, cinnamon, butter, and sugar. Set aside.

To make the cake

1. Preheat the oven to 350f. Spray a 9-inch square pan with cooking spray. Set aside.

2. In a large bowl, stir together the pastry flour, oat flour, sugar, and baking powder.

3. Add the egg, milk, butter, and lemon peel, and stir until there are no dry spots.

4. Stir in the blueberries, and gently mix until incorporated. Press the batter into the prepared pan, using a spoon to flatten it into the dish.

5. Sprinkle the topping over the cake.

6. Bake for 40 to 45 minutes, until a toothpick inserted into the cake comes out clean, and serve.

Nutrition: calories: 177; total fat: 7g; saturated fat: 3g; protein: 4g; carbs: 26g; sugar: 9g; fiber: 3g; cholesterol: 26mg; sodium: 39mg

Whole-grain pancakes

Preparation time: 10 minutes

Cooking time: 15 minutes

Servings: 4 to 6

Ingredients:

- 2 cups whole-wheat pastry flour

- 4 teaspoons baking powder

- 2 teaspoons ground cinnamon

- 1/2 teaspoon salt

- 2 cups skim milk, plus more as needed

- 2 large eggs

- 1 tablespoon honey

- Nonstick cooking spray

- Maple syrup, for serving

- Fresh fruit, for serving

Directions:

1. In a large bowl, stir together the flour, baking powder, cinnamon, and salt.

2. Add the milk, eggs, and honey, and stir well to combine. If needed, add more milk, 1 tablespoon at a time, until there are no dry spots and you has a pourable batter.

3. Heat a large skillet over medium-high heat, and spray it with cooking spray.

4. Using a ¼-cup measuring cup, scoop 2 or 3 pancakes into the skillet at a time. Cook for a couple of minutes, until bubbles form on the surface of the pancakes, flip, and cook for 1 to 2 minutes more, until golden brown and cooked through. Repeat with the remaining batter.

5. Serve topped with maple syrup or fresh fruit.

Nutrition: calories: 392; total fat: 4g; saturated fat: 1g; protein: 15g; carbs: 71g; sugar: 11g; fiber: 9g; cholesterol: 95mg; sodium: 396mg

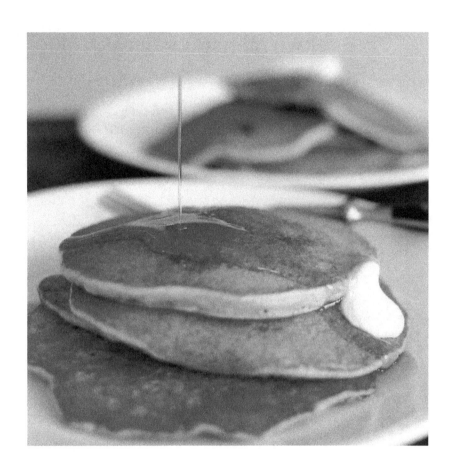

Buckwheat grouts breakfast bowl

Preparation time: 5 minutes, plus overnight to soak
Cooking time: 10 to 12 minutes
Servings: 4
Ingredients:

- 3 cups skim milk

- 1 cup buckwheat grouts

- ¼ cup chia seeds

- 2 teaspoons vanilla extract

- 1/2 teaspoon ground cinnamon

- Pinch salt

- 1 cup water

- 1/2 cup unsalted pistachios

- 2 cups sliced fresh strawberries

- ¼ cup cacao nibs (optional)

Directions:

1. In a large bowl, stir together the milk, groats, chia seeds, vanilla, cinnamon, and salt. Cover and refrigerate overnight.

2. The next morning, transfer the soaked mixture to a medium pot and add the water. Bring to a boil over medium-high heat, reduce the heat to maintain a simmer, and cook for 10 to 12 minutes, until the buckwheat is tender and thickened.

3. Transfer to bowls and serve, topped with the pistachios, strawberries, and cacao nibs (if using).

Nutrition: calories: 340; total fat: 8g; saturated fat: 1g; protein: 15g; carbs: 52g; sugar: 14g; fiber: 10g; cholesterol: 4mg; sodium: 140mg

Peach muesli bake

Preparation time: 10 minutes

Cooking time: 40 minutes

Servings: 8

Ingredients:

- Nonstick cooking spray

- 2 cups skim milk

- 11/2 cups rolled oats

- 1/2 cup chopped walnuts

- 1 large egg

- 2 tablespoons maple syrup

- 1 teaspoon ground cinnamon

- 1 teaspoon baking powder

- 1/2 teaspoon salt

- 2 to 3 peaches, sliced

Directions:

1. Preheat the oven to 375f. Spray a 9-inch square baking dish with cooking spray. Set aside.

2. In a large bowl, stir together the milk, oats, walnuts, egg, maple syrup, cinnamon, baking powder, and salt. Spread half the mixture in the prepared baking dish.

3. Place half the peaches in a single layer across the oat mixture.

4. Spread the remaining oat mixture over the top. Add the remaining peaches in a thin layer over the oats. Bake for 35 to 40 minutes, uncovered, until thickened and browned.

5. Cut into 8 squares and serve warm.

Nutrition: calories: 138; total fat: 3g; saturated fat: 1g; protein: 6g; carbs: 22g; sugar: 10g; fiber: 3g; cholesterol: 24mg; sodium: 191mg

Steel-cut oatmeal bowl with fruit and nuts

Preparation time: 5 minutes

Cooking time: 20 minutes

Servings: 4

Ingredients:

- 1 cup steel-cut oats

- 2 cups almond milk

- ¾ cup water

- 1 teaspoon ground cinnamon

- ¼ teaspoon salt

- 2 cups chopped fresh fruit, such as blueberries, strawberries, raspberries, or peaches

- 1/2 cup chopped walnuts

- ¼ cup chia seeds

Directions:

1. In a medium saucepan over medium-high heat, combine the oats, almond milk, water, cinnamon, and salt. Bring to a boil, reduce the heat to low, and simmer for 15 to 20 minutes, until the oats are softened and thickened.

2. Top each bowl with 1/2 cup of fresh fruit, 2 tablespoons of walnuts, and 1 tablespoon of chia seeds before serving.

Nutrition: calories: 288; total fat: 11g; saturated fat: 1g; protein: 10g; carbs: 38g; sugar: 7g; fiber: 10g; cholesterol: 0mg; sodium: 329mg

Whole-grain dutch baby pancake

Preparation time: 5 minutes

Cooking time: 25 minutes

Servings: 4

Ingredients:

- 2 tablespoons coconut oil

- 1/2 cup whole-wheat flour

- ¼ cup skim milk

- 3 large eggs

- 1 teaspoon vanilla extract

- 1/2 teaspoon baking powder

- ¼ teaspoon salt

- ¼ teaspoon ground cinnamon

- Powdered sugar, for dusting

Directions:

1. Preheat the oven to 400f.

2. Put the coconut oil in a medium oven-safe skillet, and place the skillet in the oven to melt the oil while it preheats.

3. In a blender, combine the flour, milk, eggs, vanilla, baking powder, salt, and cinnamon. Process until smooth.

4. Carefully remove the skillet from the oven and tilt to spread the oil around evenly.

5. Pour the batter into the skillet and return it to the oven for 23 to 25 minutes, until the pancake puffs and lightly browns.

6. Remove, dust lightly with powdered sugar, cut into 4 wedges, and serve.

Nutrition: calories: 195; total fat: 11g; saturated fat: 7g; protein: 8g; carbs: 16g; sugar: 1g; fiber: 2g; cholesterol: 140mg; sodium: 209mg

Mushroom, zucchini, and onion frittata

Preparation time: 10 minutes

Cooking time: 20 minutes

Servings: 4

Ingredients:

- 1 tablespoon extra-virgin olive oil

- 1/2 onion, chopped

- 1 medium zucchini, chopped

- 11/2 cups sliced mushrooms

- 6 large eggs, beaten

- 2 tablespoons skim milk

- Salt

- Freshly ground black pepper

- 1 ounce feta cheese, crumbled

Directions:

1. Preheat the oven to 400f.

2. In a medium oven-safe skillet over medium-high heat, heat the olive oil.

3. Add the onion and sauté for 3 to 5 minutes, until translucent.

4. Add the zucchini and mushrooms, and cook for 3 to 5 more minutes, until the vegetables are tender.

5. Meanwhile, in a small bowl, whisk the eggs, milk, salt, and pepper. Pour the mixture into the skillet, stirring to combine, and transfer the skillet to the oven. Cook for 7 to 9 minutes, until set.

6. Sprinkle with the feta cheese, and cook for 1 to 2 minutes more, until heated through.

7. Remove, cut into 4 wedges, and serve.

Nutrition: calories: 178; total fat: 13g; saturated fat: 4g; protein: 12g; carbs: 5g; sugar: 3g; fiber: 1g; cholesterol: 285mg; sodium: 234mg

Spinach and cheese quiche

Preparation time: 10 minutes, plus 10 minutes to rest
Cooking time: 50 minutes
Servings: 4 to 6
Ingredients:

- Nonstick cooking spray

- 8 ounces yukon gold potatoes, shredded

- 1 tablespoon plus 2 teaspoons extra-virgin olive oil, divided

- 1 teaspoon salt, divided

- Freshly ground black pepper

- 1 onion, finely chopped

- 1 (10-ounce) bag fresh spinach

- 4 large eggs

- 1/2 cup skim milk

- 1 ounce gruyère cheese, shredded

Directions:

1. Preheat the oven to 350f. Spray a 9-inch pie dish with cooking spray. Set aside.

2. In a small bowl, toss the potatoes with 2 teaspoons of olive oil, 1/2 teaspoon of salt, and season with pepper. Press the potatoes into the bottom and sides of the pie dish to form a thin, even layer. Bake for 20 minutes, until golden brown. Remove from the oven and set aside to cool.

3. In a large skillet over medium-high heat, heat the remaining 1 tablespoon of olive oil.

4. Add the onion and sauté for 3 to 5 minutes, until softened.

5. By handfuls, add the spinach, stirring between each addition, until it just starts to wilt before adding more. Cook for about 1 minute, until it cooks down.

6. In a medium bowl, whisk the eggs and milk. Add the gruyère, and season with the remaining 1/2 teaspoon of salt and some pepper. Fold the eggs into the spinach. Pour the mixture into the pie dish and bake for 25 minutes, until the eggs are set.

7. Let rest for 10 minutes before serving.

Nutrition: calories: 445; total fat: 14g; saturated fat: 4g; protein: 19g; carbs: 68g; sugar: 6g; fiber: 7g; cholesterol: 193mg; sodium: 773mg

Lunch

Lemony Salmon Burgers

Preparation Time: 10 Minutes

Cooking Time: 10 Minutes

Servings: 4

Ingredients

- 2 (3-oz) cans boneless, skinless pink salmon
- 1/4 cup panko breadcrumbs
- 4 tsp. lemon juice
- 1/4 cup red bell pepper
- 1/4 cup sugar-free yogurt
- 1 egg
- 2 (1.5-oz) whole wheat hamburger toasted buns

Directions

1. Mix drained and flaked salmon, finely-chopped bell pepper, panko breadcrumbs.

2. Combine 2 tbsp. cup sugar-free yogurt, 3 tsp. fresh lemon juice, and egg in a bowl. Shape mixture into 2 (3-inch) patties, bake on the skillet over medium heat 4 to 5 Minutes per side.

3. Stir together 2 tbsp. sugar-free yogurt and 1 tsp. lemon juice; spread over bottom halves of buns.

4. Top each with 1 patty, and cover with bun tops.

This dish is very mouth-watering!

Nutrition:

Calories 131 / Protein 12 / Fat 1 g / Carbs 19 g

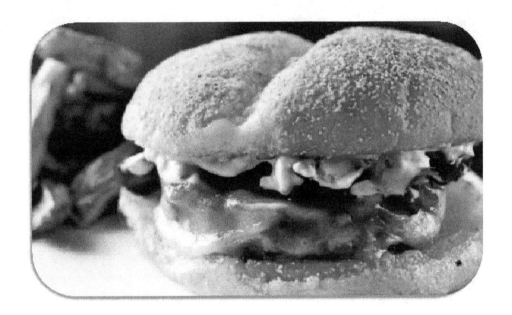

Caprese Turkey Burgers

Preparation Time 10 Minutes

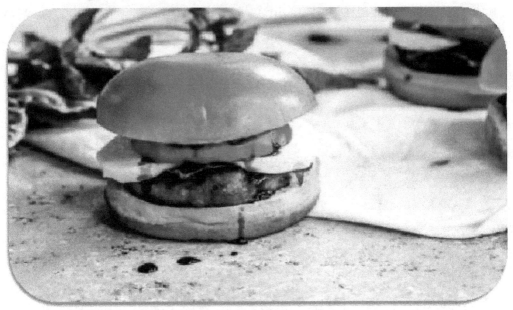

Cooking Time: 10 Minutes

Servings: 4

Ingredients

- 1/2 lb. 93% lean ground turkey
- 2 (1,5-oz) whole wheat hamburger buns (toasted)
- 1/4 cup shredded mozzarella cheese (part-skim)
- 1 egg
- 1 big tomato
- 1 small clove garlic
- 4 large basil leaves

- 1/8 tsp. salt
- 1/8 tsp. pepper

Directions

1. Combine turkey, white egg, Minced garlic, salt, and pepper (mix until combined);
2. Shape into 2 cutlets. Put cutlets into a skillet; cook 5 to 7 Minutes per side.
3. Top cutlets properly with cheese and sliced tomato at the end of cooking.
4. Put 1 cutlet on the bottom of each bun.
5. Top each patty with 2 basil leaves. Cover with bun tops.

My guests enjoy this dish every time they visit my home.

Nutrition:

Calories 180 / Protein 7 g / Fat 4 g / Carbs 20 g

Pasta Salad

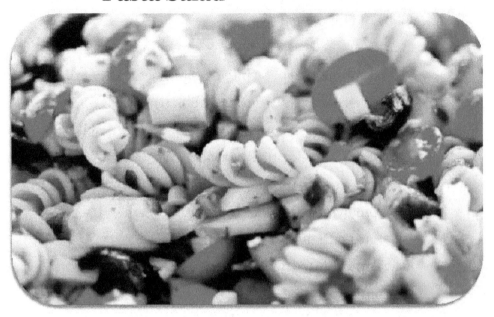

Preparation Time: 15 Minutes

Cooking Time: 15 Minutes

Servings: 4

Ingredients

- 8 oz. whole-wheat pasta
- 2 tomatoes
- 1 (5-oz) pkg spring mix
- 9 slices bacon
- 1/3 cup mayonnaise (reduced-fat)
- 1 tbsp. Dijon mustard
- 3 tbsp. apple cider vinegar
- 1/4 tsp. salt

- 1/2 tsp. pepper

Directions

1. Cook pasta.
2. Chilled pasta, chopped tomatoes and spring mix in a bowl.
3. Crumble cooked bacon over pasta.
4. Combine mayonnaise, mustard, vinegar, salt and pepper in a small bowl.
5. Pour dressing over pasta, stirring to coat.

Understanding diabetes is the first step in curing.

Nutrition:

Calories 200 / Protein 15 g / Fat 3 g / Carbs 6 g

Conclusion

I hope you have enjoyed these recipes as much as I have. Life with diabetes should not be hard. It is not the end—it is the beginning. With healthy dietary management, you can lead a life free from the negative effects of high (or low) blood sugar levels.

With the knowledge I have shared, you now know why you may have become diabetic, you know what this means, and now, you also know how to manage it. You are armed with resources, apps, and recipes to help you along this lifelong journey. Food is not your enemy; it's your friend.

Cook your way to health and vitality with these recipes and tips. Good things are made to share, so please help a friend find out about this way of life. Call them over for a meal, talk about diabetes, and let's help create awareness as we feast on every delectable spoonful of diabetic cooking made easy.

The warning symptoms of diabetes type 1 are the same as type 2, however, in type 1, these signs and symptoms tend to occur slowly over a period of months or years, making it harder to spot and recognize. Some of these symptoms can even occur after the disease has progressed.

Each disorder has risk factors that when found in an individual, favor the development of the disease. Diabetes is no different. Here are some of the risk factors for developing diabetes.

Having a Family History of Diabetes

Usually having a family member, especially first-degree relatives could be an indicator that you are at risk to develop diabetes. Your risk of developing diabetes is about 15% if you have one parent with diabetes while it is 75% if both your parents have diabetes.

Having Prediabetes

Being pre-diabetic means that you have higher than normal blood glucose levels. However, they are not high enough to be diagnosed as type 2 diabetes. Having pre-diabetes is a risk factor for developing type 2 diabetes as well as other conditions such as cardiac conditions. Since there are no symptoms or signs for prediabetes, it is often a latent condition that is discovered accidentally during routine investigations of blood glucose levels or when investigating other conditions.

Being Obese or Overweight

Your metabolism, fat stores and eating habits when you are overweight or above the healthy weight range contributes to abnormal metabolism pathways that put you at risk for developing diabetes type 2. There have been consistent research results of the obvious link between developing diabetes and being obese.

Having a Sedentary Lifestyle

Having a lifestyle where you are mostly physically inactive predisposes you to a lot of conditions including diabetes type 2. That is because being physically inactive causes you to develop obesity or become overweight. Moreover, you don't burn any excess sugars that you ingest which can lead you to become prediabetic and eventually diabetic.

Having Gestational Diabetes Developing gestational diabetes which is diabetes that occurred due to pregnancy (and often disappears after pregnancy) is a risk factor for developing diabetes at some point.

Ethnicity

Belonging to certain ethnic groups such as Middle Eastern, South Asian or Indian background. Studies of statistics have revealed that the prevalence of diabetes type 2 in these ethnic groups is high. If you come from any of these ethnicities, this puts you at risk of developing diabetes type 2 yourself.

Having Hypertension

Studies have shown an association between having hypertension and having an increased risk of developing diabetes. If you have hypertension, you should not leave it uncontrolled.

Extremes of Age

Diabetes can occur at any age. However, being too young or too old means your body is not in its best form and therefore, this increases the risk of developing diabetes.

That sounds scary. However, diabetes only occurs with the presence of a combination of these risk factors. Most of the risk factors can be minimized by taking action. For example, developing a more active lifestyle, taking care of your habits and attempting to lower your blood glucose sugar by restricting your sugar intake. If you start to notice you are prediabetic or getting overweight, etc., there is always something you can do to modify the situation. Recent studies show that developing healthy eating habits and following diets that are low in carbs, losing excess weight and leading an active lifestyle can help to protect you from developing diabetes, especially diabetes type 2, by minimizing the risk factors of developing the disorder.

You can also have an oral glucose tolerance test in which you will have a fasting glucose test first and then you will be given a sugary drink and then having your blood glucose tested 2 hours after that to see how your body responds to glucose meals. In healthy individuals, the blood glucose should drop again 2 hours post sugary meals due to the action of insulin.

Another indicative test is the HbA1C. This test reflects the average of your blood glucose level over the last 2 to 3 months. It is also a test to see how well you manage your diabetes.

People with diabetes type 1 require compulsory insulin shots to control their diabetes because they have no other option. People with diabetes type 2 can regulate their diabetes with healthy eating and regular physical activity although they may require some glucose-lowering medications that can be in tablet form or in the form of an injection.

All the above goes in the direction that you need to avoid a starchy diet because of its tendency to raise the blood glucose levels. Too many carbohydrates can lead to insulin sensitivity and pancreatic fatigue; as well as weight gain with all its associated risk factors for cardiovascular disease and hypertension. The solution is to lower your sugar intake, therefore, decrease your body's need for insulin and increase the burning of fat in your body.

When your body is low on sugars, it will be forced to use a subsequent molecule to burn for energy, in that case, this will be fat. The burning of fat will lead you to lose weight.

I hope you have learned something!